I Heard You Wanna Celebrate The Holidays

Tiana Hampton

I HEARD YOU WANNA CELEBRATE THE HOLIDAYS

Paperback ISBN: 978-1-965593-71-4

Published by Cornerstone Publishing

A Division of Cornerstone Creativity Group LLC
Info@thecornerstonepublishers.com
www.thecornerstonepublishers.com

Author's Contact

To book the author to speak at your next event or to order bulk copies of this book, please, use the information below:

tianahampton91@gmail.com

Printed in the United States of America.

A Note to My Readers

Thank you for picking up this little piece of holiday magic. This book was created straight from my bar to your home, with love, glitter, and a splash of mischief.

The holidays can be chaotic, emotional, hilarious, and unforgettable all at the same time. My hope is that every recipe in here brings you a moment of joy, a cute lil escape, or the perfect excuse to toast to something worth celebrating. Whether you're mixing for a crowd, sipping solo in fuzzy socks, or showing off your bartending skills at the family function, you deserve a drink that feels as good as it tastes.

Cheers to love, life, and the kind of nights that turn into stories. Now grab your shaker, cue the holiday playlist, and let's celebrate the season together.

With Love,

Tati

Contents

Thanksgiving

My Thanksgiving Story

Thanksgiving has always been the true beginning of the holidays for my family. When I was little, everything started at my Granny Dot's house. That was the heart of our world. I can still taste her dressing like it's sitting on the table right in front of me. The kind of flavor you don't just remember — it stays with you.

Those gatherings at Granny Dot's weren't just meals. They were the moments that shaped us. The laughter in the kitchen, the chairs scraping the floor as more cousins showed up, the way everyone squeezed around the table even when there wasn't enough room.

As we got older, Thanksgiving started branching out into Saturday potlucks that led us right into the Christmas season. But no matter how life changed,

Granny Dot's house was our anchor. We always had Sunday dinners, but Thanksgiving was the one day everybody came together — no excuses, no missing faces, just love filling every corner.

For me, Thanksgiving will always mean warmth, togetherness, and the comfort of knowing you belong to something bigger than yourself. And that's the energy I wanted to bring into the cocktails in this chapter: cozy, familiar, and made with love.

Pumpkin Spice & Everything Nice Espresso Martini

1.5 oz vodka

1.5 oz pumpkin spice syrup

1.5 oz coffee liqueur

1.5 oz expresso

Powdered cinnamon and coffee beans for garnish

**Add all ingredients to a cocktail shaker and shake for a couple of seconds. Add ice and shake again. Strain into chilled coupe glass. Please note not adding shaking drink contents first before ice will create the “forth effect”. Garnish with powdered cinnamon and coffee beans.

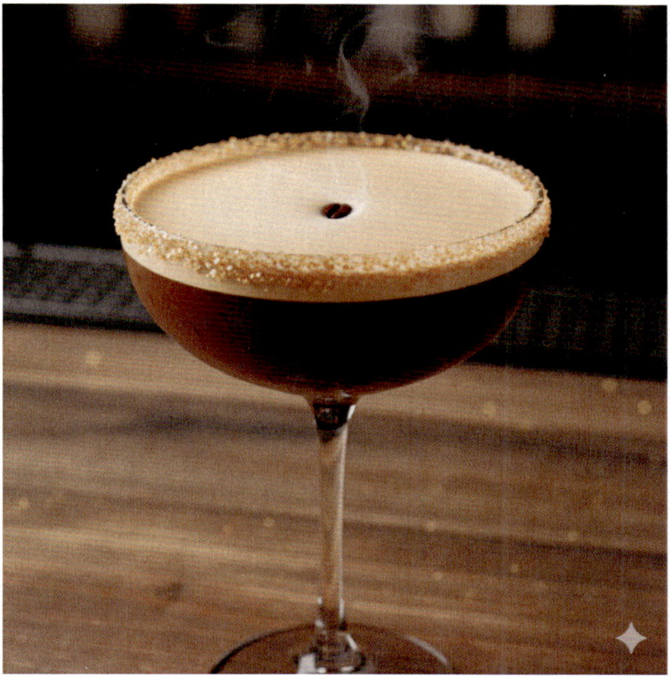

Spiked Sweet Potato Pie

2 oz Vanilla Vodka

1.5 oz Sweet Potato Puree

1 oz Triple Sec

1 tsp vanilla extract

Brown sugar for martini glass rim

**Add all ingredients to a cocktail shaker and shake for a couple of seconds. Add ice and shake again. Strain into brown sugared rim martini glass. Please note not adding shaking drink contents first before ice will create the "forth effect".

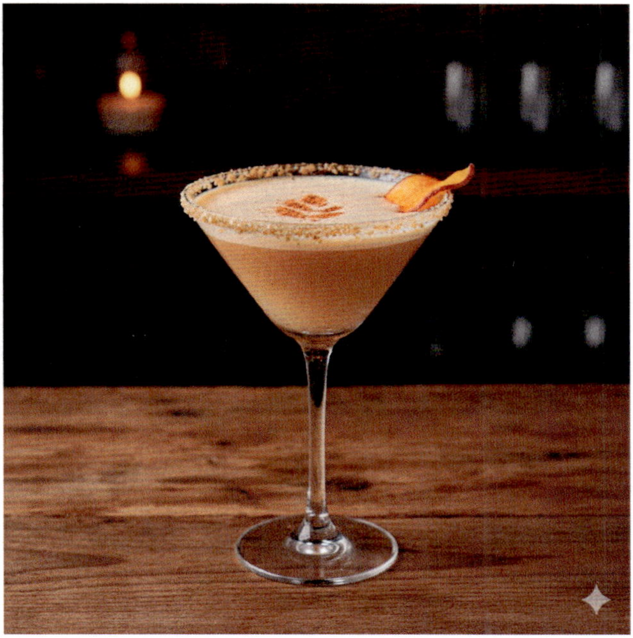

Thankful, Tipsy, & Thriving (Makes 6 Servings)

1 Bottle White Wine

1 Cup Muddled Cranberries

½ Cup of Apple Cider

¼ Cup of Simple Syrup

½ Cup of Brandy

1 cup of diced apple

½ Cup of Cranberries

2 Cinnamon Sticks

1 Piece of Fresh Sliced Ginger

1 Sliced Orange

Add ingredients to a pitcher with ice. Stir well. Serve in rocks glass with ice. Garnish with orange slices, cranberries, and apples.

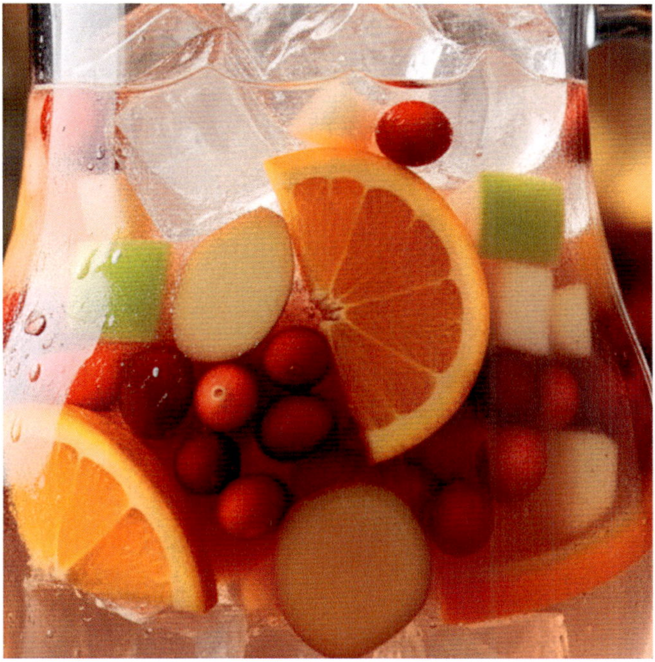

The Autumn Affair

2 oz cognac

2 oz apple cider

1 oz Cointreau

½ oz Lemon Juice

1 oz Grand Marnier

**Add all ingredients to a cocktail shaker with ice. Shake for a couple of seconds. Pour contents into a sugared rimmed coupe glass. Add a fresh apple slice and a lemon wedge as garnish.

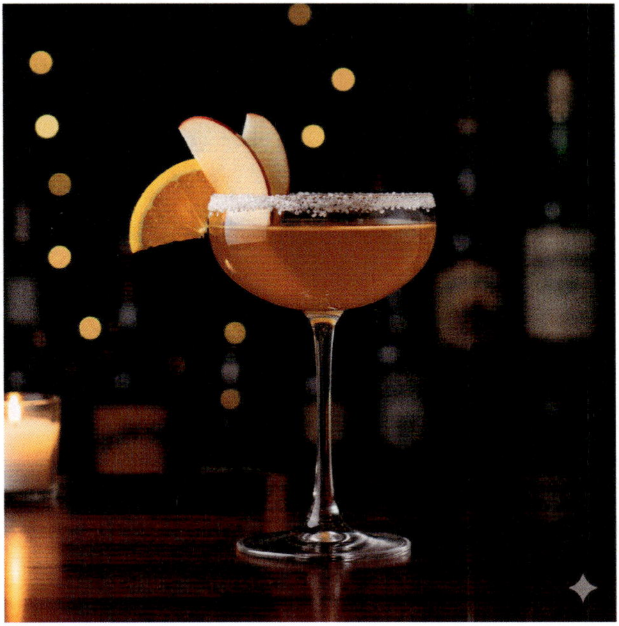

Cozy Pear Mule

2 oz whiskey

2 oz Pear Puree

½ Lime Juice

Ginger Beer

**In a copper mug, add ingredients with ice. Top off with ginger beer. Garnish with lime wheel and fresh diced pears.

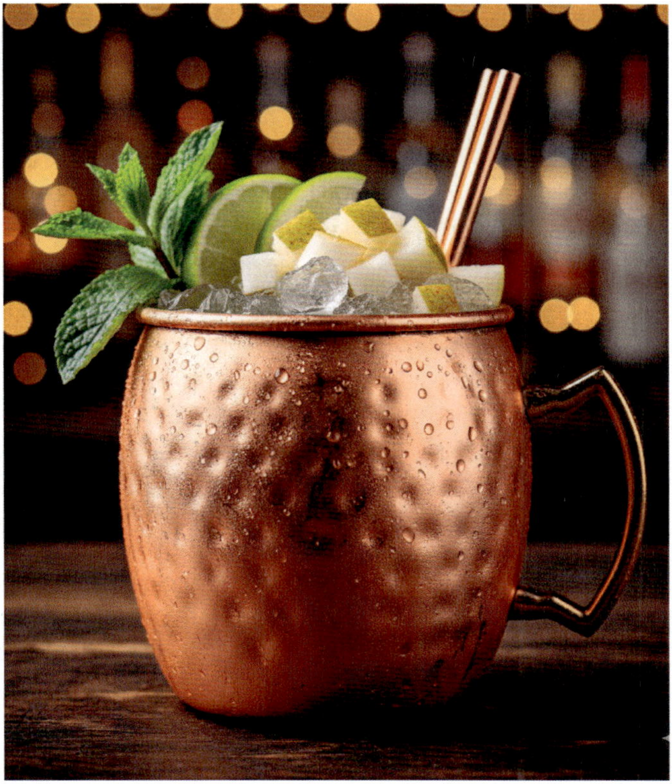

Cuffing Season Margarita

2 oz Reposado Tequila

2 oz Lime Juice

2 oz Hot Honey

½ oz Triple Sec

¾ Orange Juice

**Add all ingredients to a cocktail shaker with ice. Shake for a couple of seconds. Pour contents into a Tajin rimmed glass over ice. Add Lime Wheel as garnish.

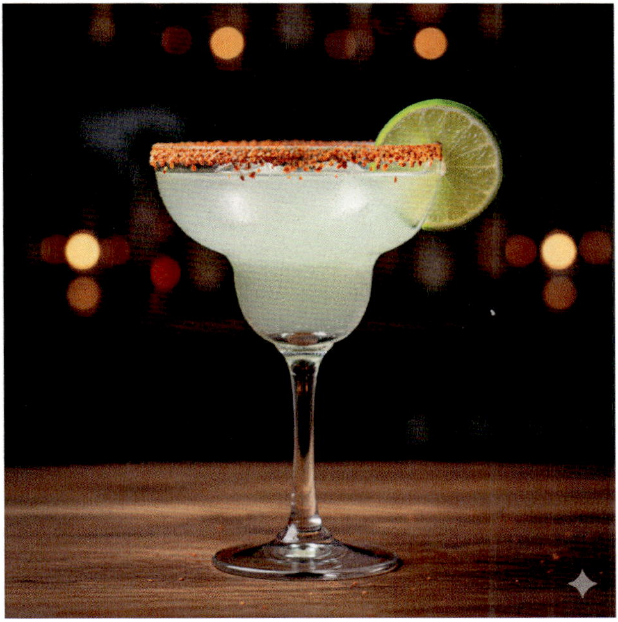

Falling for You Fizz Mocktail

3 oz White Grape Juice

3 oz Apple Juice

½ oz Lemon juice

Ginger Beer

**Add all ingredients to a cocktail shaker with ice. Shake for a couple of seconds. Pour content into glass with ice. Top off with ginger beer. Garnish with apple slices. *Turn this into a "cocktail" by adding 2 oz of gin.*

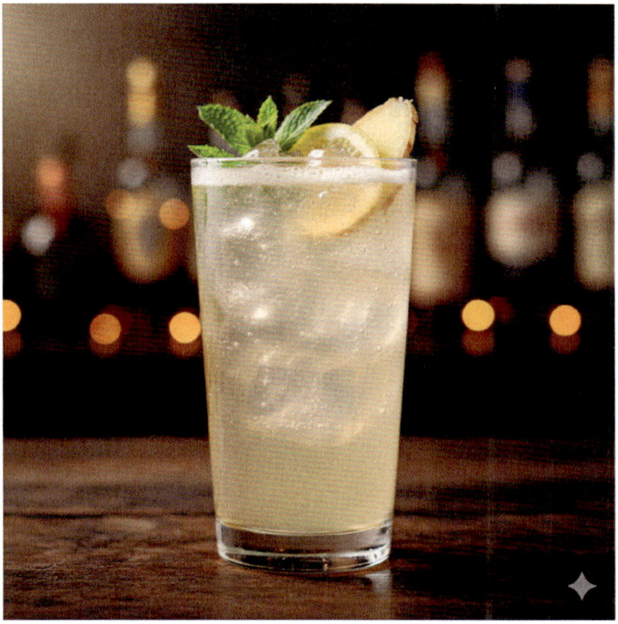

Grateful and Gorgeous

2 oz Gin

2 oz Triple Sec

1 oz Lemon Juice

2 oz Fig Puree

**Add all ingredients to a cocktail shaker with ice. Shake for a couple of seconds. Pour contents into a chilled sugared rimmed martini glass. Add a fresh fig slice and a lemon wedge as garnish.

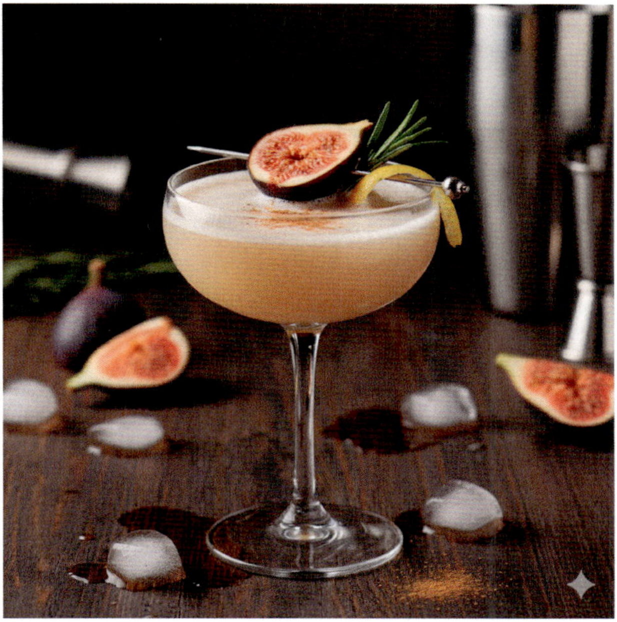

Friendsgiving Fizz

½ oz Carmel Vodka

2 oz of Apple Juice

Champagne

**In a champagne flute add caramel vodka and apple juice. Top off with Champagne.

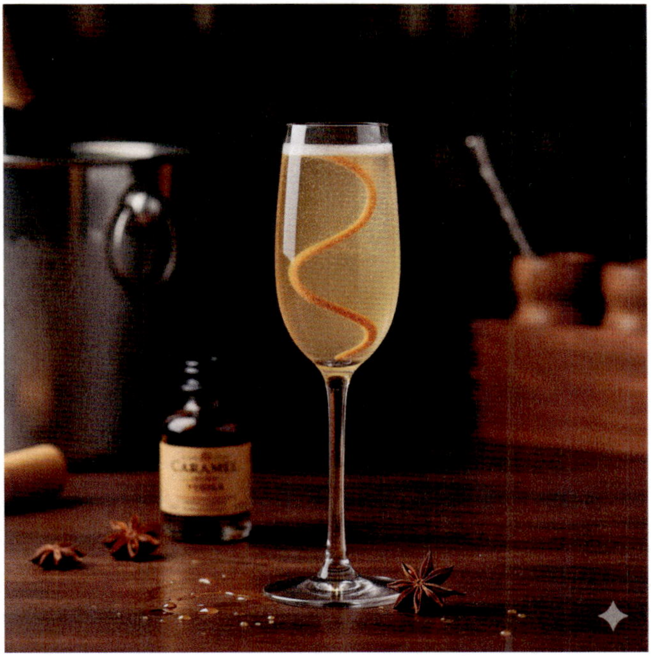

Feast Mode Mocktail Punch (Serves 6)

4 Cups of Apple Cider

2 Cups of Cranberry Juice

1 Cup of Orange Juice

½ cup of Pear Juice

3 Cinnamon Sticks

**Add ingredients to a large pitcher. Add ice and stir. Add fresh apple and orange slices. *Turn this into a cocktail by adding ½ cup of Rum.*

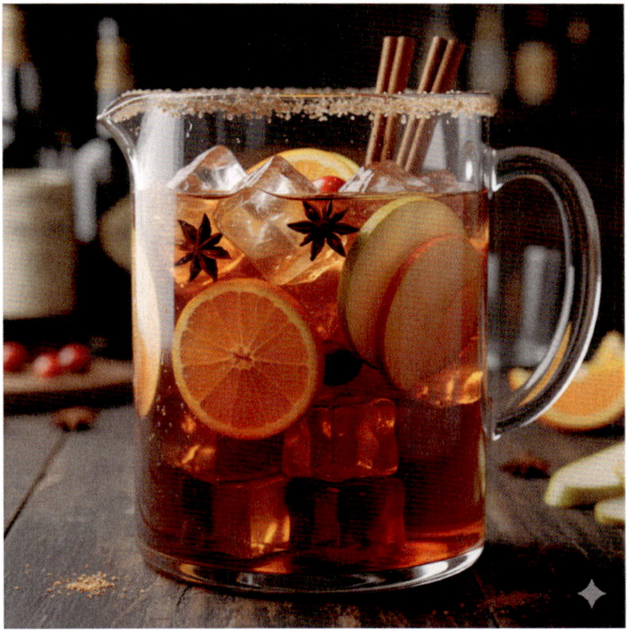

Christmas

My Christmas Story

My family has always done Christmas big. Like... BIG big. Just like Thanksgiving, everything started at Granny Dot's house. I'll never forget those mornings filled with every breakfast food you could think of — even Kaboom cereal — and the sound of all of us kids running through the house like pure chaos wrapped in holiday spirit. My cousins and I were all close in age, so whatever one of us got, you could bet the other two had it too. We were a little squad, and Christmas felt like our own adventure every single year.

At home, my mom made the holidays magical in her own way. Even working long shifts as a nurse, she always made sure Christmas felt special to us. She used to tell us that Santa loved chocolate cake and Pepsi, and we believed it with our whole hearts. I still remember waking up in our matching Christmas pajamas to the smell of bacon and hot cocoa drifting through the house. Those mornings felt like comfort, love, and excitement all in one.

As the years passed, Christmas shifted to my aunt's house. Now it's the next generation — including my own kid — running around, playing games, exchanging gifts, and creating their own memories in the same spirit we grew up with. Watching them has a way of making everything come full circle.

Christmas has always meant family, joy, and a warmth that settles deep in your soul. That feeling is exactly what inspired the Christmas cocktails in this book. Every recipe in this section carries a little piece of those memories — the coziness of hot cocoa in the morning, the sweetness of childhood excitement, the comfort of family, and the sparkle of creating new traditions. These cocktails are my way of honoring the magic I grew up with and sharing that same holiday glow with you.

The Claus Effect

2 oz Vodka

3 oz Cranberry Juice

Sparking Rose

Fresh Cranberries

**Add vodka, cranberry with ice to a rocks glass. Top off with sparkling rose. Garnish with 3-4 cranberries.

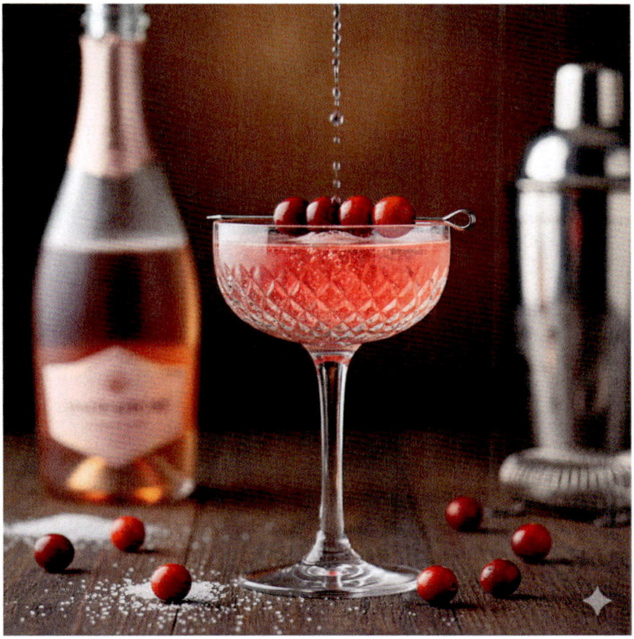

HO HO Hold My Drink Martini

1.5 oz Vodka

1.5 oz Cointreau

1.5 oz Cranberry Juice

1.5 oz Pomegranate Juice

**Add all ingredients to a cocktail shaker with ice. Shake for a couple of seconds. Pour contents into a chilled sugared rimmed martini glass. Garnish with fresh cranberries and rosemary sprig.

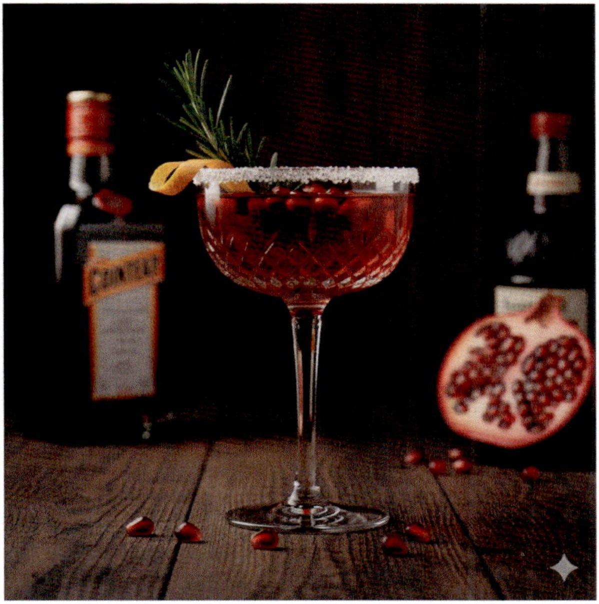

Naughty But Nice Margarita

1.5 oz Tequila

½ oz Cointreau

1.5 oz Cranberry Juice

1 oz Lime Juice

**Add all ingredients to a cocktail shaker with ice. Shake for a couple of seconds. Pour contents into a chilled sugared rimmed or salt rimmed rocks glass. Garnish with fresh cranberries and rosemary sprig.

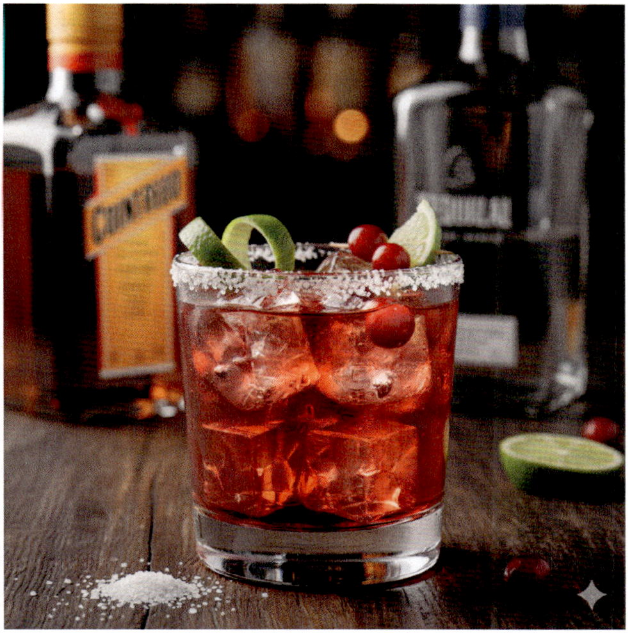

Warm Wishes and Whiskey

2 oz Whiskey

1.5 oz Cranberry Juice

2 oz Sweet and Sour Mix

½ oz Lemon Juice

**Add whiskey, cranberry juice, and lemon juice to a cocktail shaker with ice. Shake for a couple of seconds. Pour contents into a rocks glass over ice. Top off with sweet and sour mix. Garnish with lemon peel and cranberries.

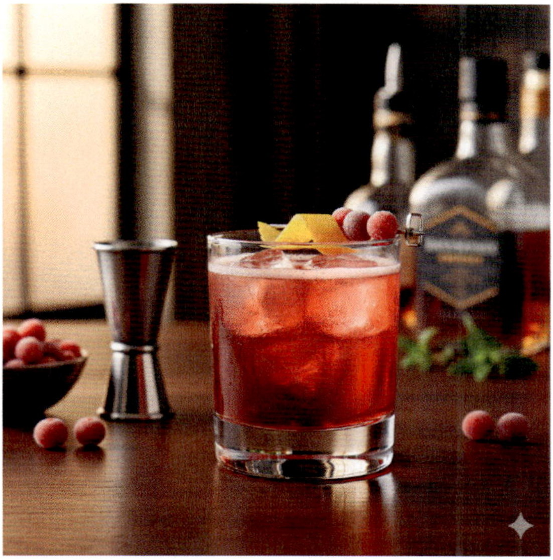

Cozy Cranberry Kiss

1.5 oz Gin

1.5 oz cranberry Juice

½ oz Simple Syrup

½ oz Lemon Juice

Champagne

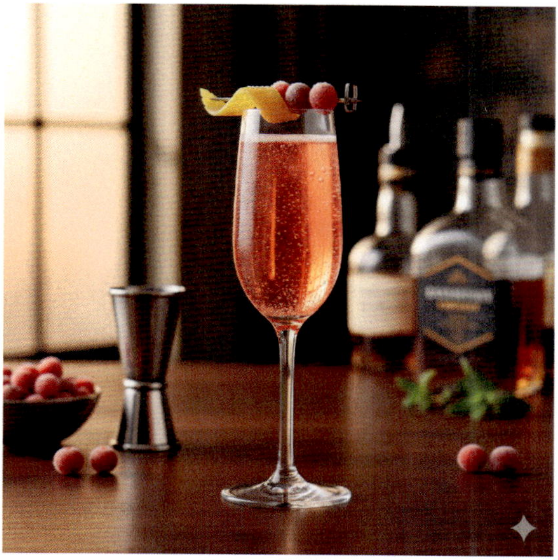

Santa Saw Me Sip

1.5 oz Vodka

½ oz St, Germain

1 oz White Cranberry Juice

½ oz Lemon Juice

**Add all ingredients to a cocktail shaker with ice. Shake for a couple of seconds. Pour contents into a chilled sugared rimmed martini glass. Garnish with 3 cranberries on a skewer dusted with sugar.

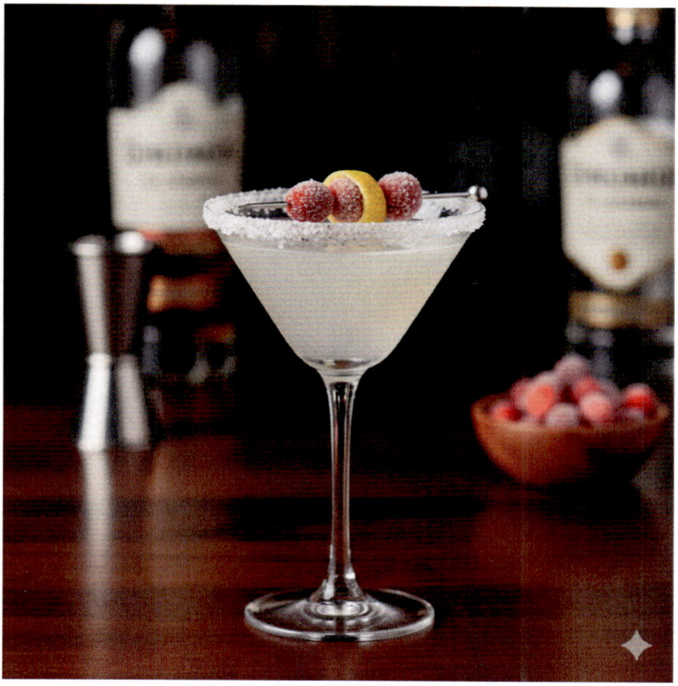

Lit-Mas Mule

1.5 oz Vodka

½ oz Peppermint Schnapps

½ oz Lime Juice

1 oz Cranberry Juice

Ginger Beer

**In a copper mug, add ingredients with ice. Top off with ginger beer. Garnish with lime wheel and cranberries.

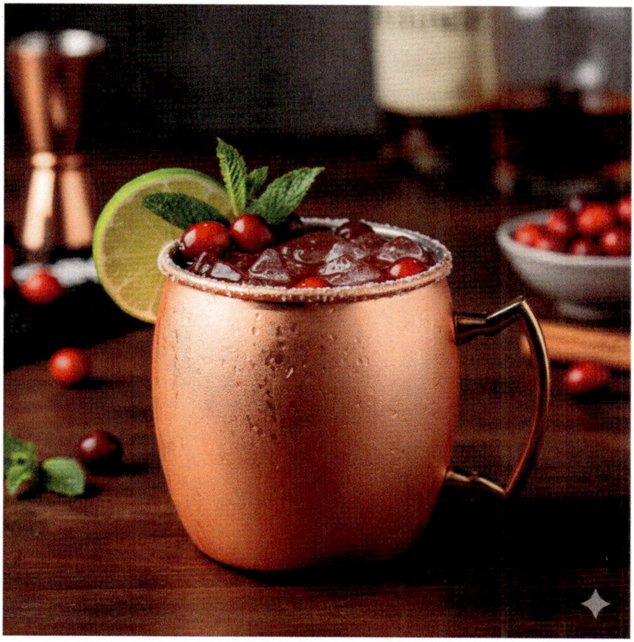

Sugar & Spice & Everything Spiked Sangria

1 Bottle of Red Wine

1 Cup of Cranberry Juice

1 Cup of Pomegranate Juice

½ Cup of Grand Marnier

½ Cup of Cinnamon Simple Syrup

**Add ingredients to a large pitcher. Add ice and stir. Add fresh apple and orange slices and cranberries.

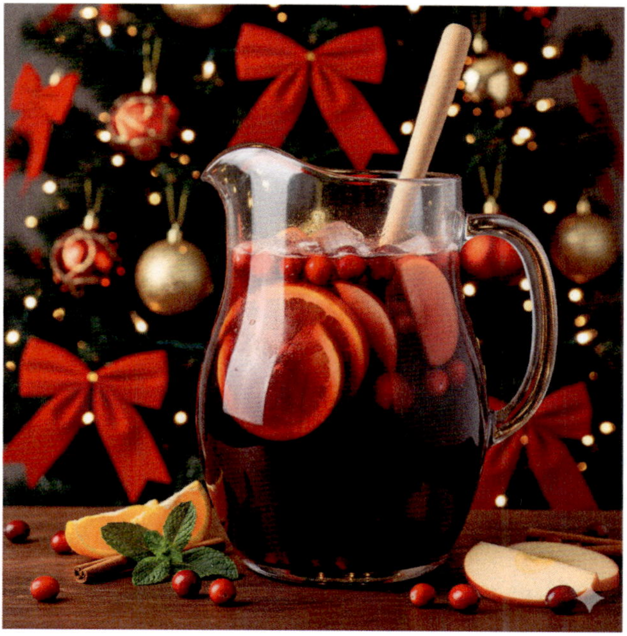

Tis the SZN to Sip

1 oz Coconut Rum

1.5 oz Midori

Lemon Lime Soda

**Add coconut rum, midori to a rocks glass with ice. Top off with lemon lime soda. Garnish with maraschino cherries.

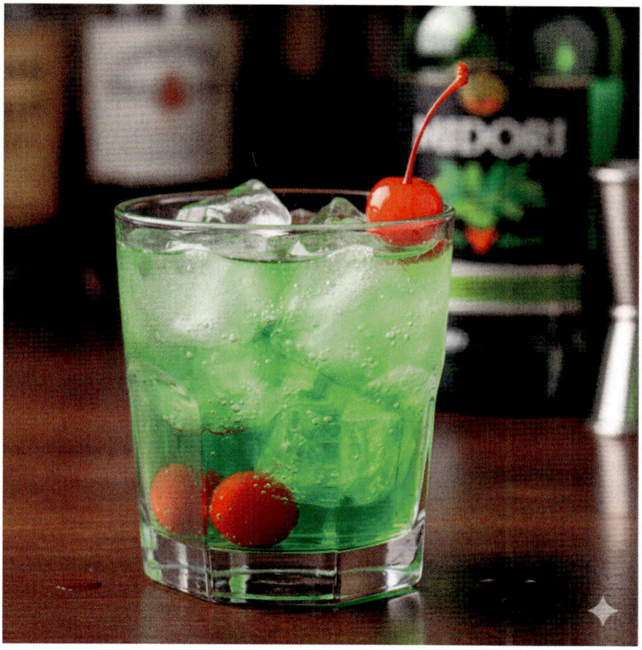

Snowglobe Babe

1.5 oz Blueberry Vodka

1 oz Blue Curacao

1 oz Cream of Coconut

½ oz Pineapple Juice

**Add all ingredients to a cocktail shaker with ice. Shake for a couple of seconds. Pour contents into a chilled coconut rimmed martini glass.

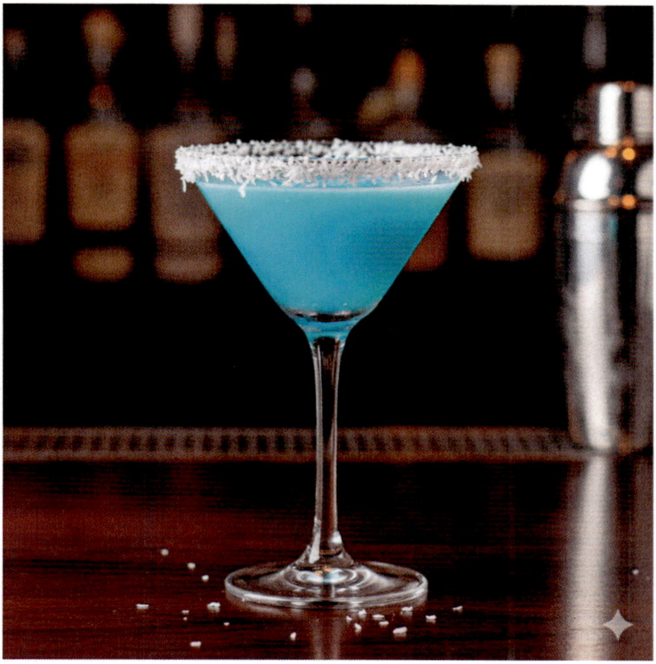

Eggnog Energy

1.5 oz Rum

½ oz Butterscotch Schnapps

3 oz of Egg Nog

**Add all ingredients to a cocktail shaker with ice. Shake for a couple of seconds. Pour contents into a rocks glass with ice. Sprinkle top with nutmeg and cinnamon.

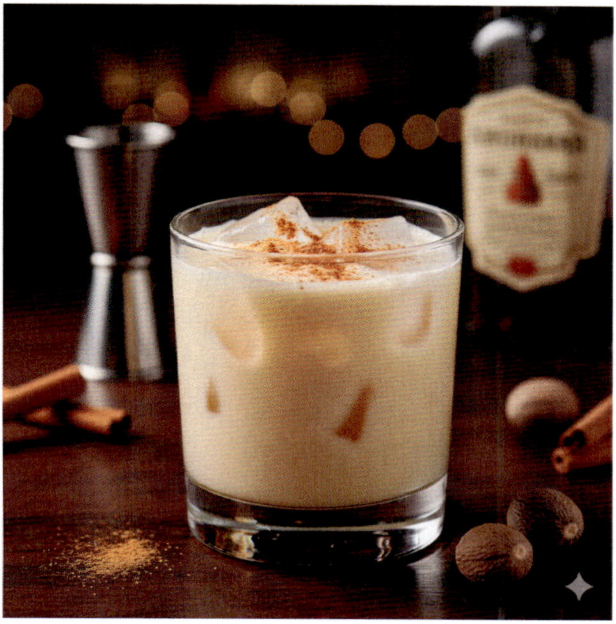

Presents & Prosecco

1 oz Peach Puree

1 oz Raspberry Puree

Sparkling Wine

**In a champagne flute add peach puree and raspberry puree. Give a quick stir. Top off with sparkling wine. Garnish with Fresh Raspberries.

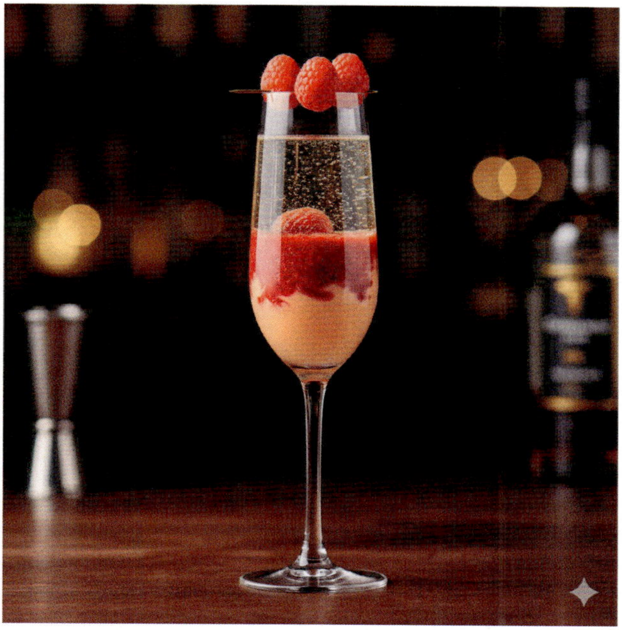

Sleigh Bells & Shots

½ oz Irish Whiskey

½ oz Peach Schnapps

½ oz Sweet and Sour Mix

½ oz Grendiene

Lemon Lime Soda

**Add irish whiskey, peach schnapps, sweet and sour mix, and lemon lime soda into a cocktail shaker with ice. Pour into shot class with grenadine as a float.

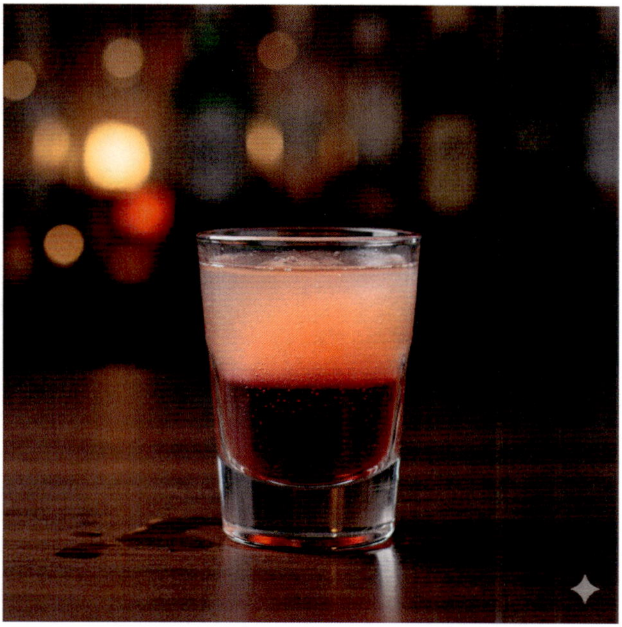

Silent Night Punch-Mocktail (Makes 6 Servings)

2 Cups Blackberry Juice

1 cup Pomegranate Juice

1 Cup of Lemon Lime Soda

**Add ingredients to a pitcher with ice. Stir well. Serve in rocks glass with ice. Garnish with blackberries and mint leaves. *Turn this into a cocktail by adding 1 cup of gin.*

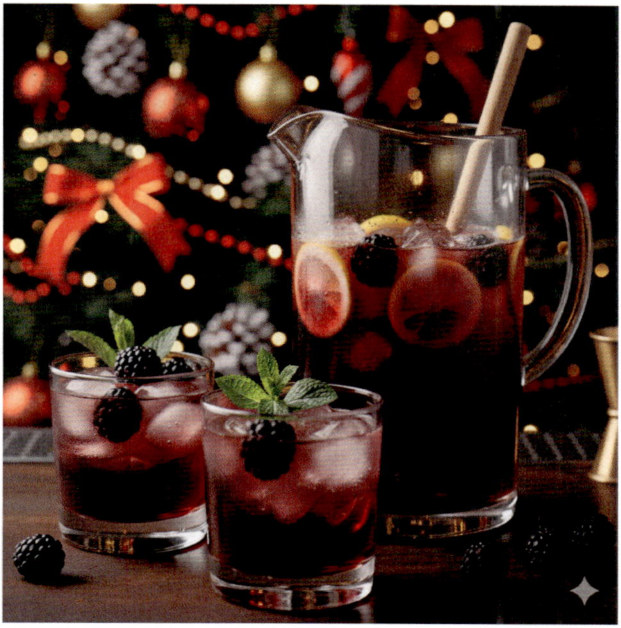

New Years Eve

My New Year's Eve Story

New Year's Eve was always a little different for my family. We didn't have one set tradition like we did for Thanksgiving or Christmas, but somehow it still felt special every year. Maybe it was the countdown energy, or the feeling that everyone everywhere was celebrating at the same time. Even without a fixed routine, there was always this quiet excitement in the air, like the whole world was taking a breath together before stepping into something new.

As I got older, New Year's Eve took on a whole different meaning for me because of the industry I work in. Being a bartender during the holidays is its own adventure. While everyone else is dressed up and ready to party, we're behind the bar shaking, pouring, smiling, keeping the night moving. I've seen couples kiss at midnight, friends; cheers to fresh starts, people crying happy tears, and strangers becoming best friends for one night. There's something magical about being part of the moment where someone decides, "This next year is going to be different."

Working New Year's Eve taught me to appreciate the celebration in a deeper way. It showed me how much a good drink, a warm atmosphere, and a little sparkle can shape the whole night. And that's exactly what inspired the New Year's Eve cocktails in this book. They're bold, bubbly, and full of energy — the kind of drinks that help you kiss the old year goodbye and welcome the new one with style.

Whether you're clinking glasses in a crowded room, hosting something cozy at home, or working the bar like I've done so many times, I hope these cocktails bring a little joy to your celebration and help you step into your next chapter feeling good.

Glitter and Goals

1.5 oz Gin

½ oz Lemon Juice

1 oz Simple Syrup

Champagne

Edible Glitter

**Add gin, edible glitter, simple syrup, and lemon juice to a cocktail shaker with ice. Shake for a couple of seconds. Pour contents into a champagne flute. Top off with champagne. Garnish with lemon twist.

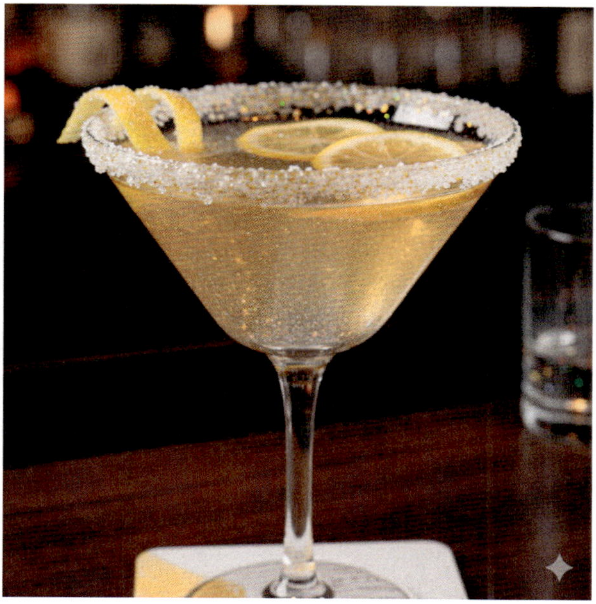

Very Berry New Year

1 oz Berry Flavored Vodka

1.5 oz Cranberry Juice

Champagne

**Add berry flavored vodka and cranberry juice to a cocktail shaker with ice. Shake for a couple of seconds. Pour contents into a champagne flute. Top off with champagne. Garnish with Lemon twist.

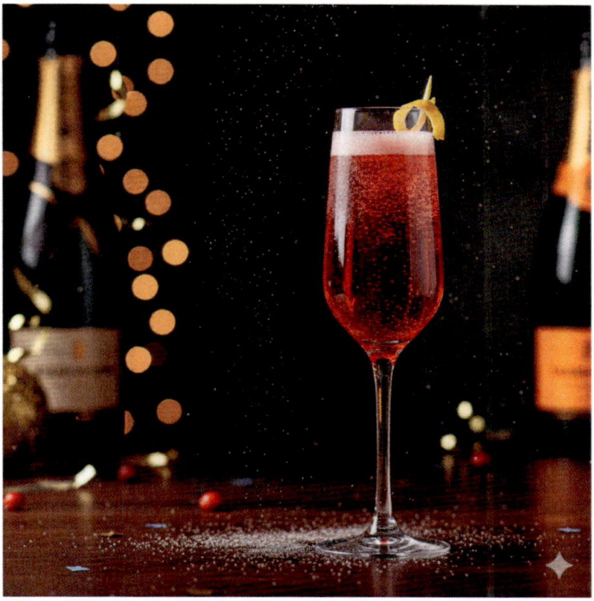

The Ball Drop Bubbly

1.5 oz Pink Whitney Vodka

2 oz White Peach Daiquiri Mix

½ Lemon Juice

Soda Water

Edible Glitter

**Add Pink Whitney Vodka, white peach daiquiri mix, lemon juice and edible glitter into a cocktail shaker with ice. Shake for a couple of seconds. Pour contents into a coupe glass. Top off with soda water. Garnish with lemon twist.

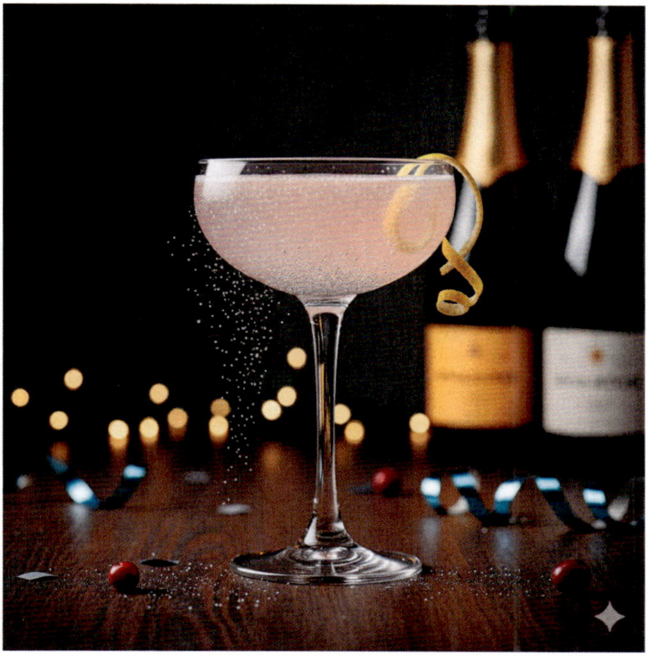

Manifest-tini

2 oz Vodka

1 oz Lemon Juice

1 oz Triple Sec

½ oz Simple Syrup

**Add all ingredients to a cocktail shaker with ice. Shake for a couple of seconds. Pour contents into a chilled sugared rimmed martini glass.

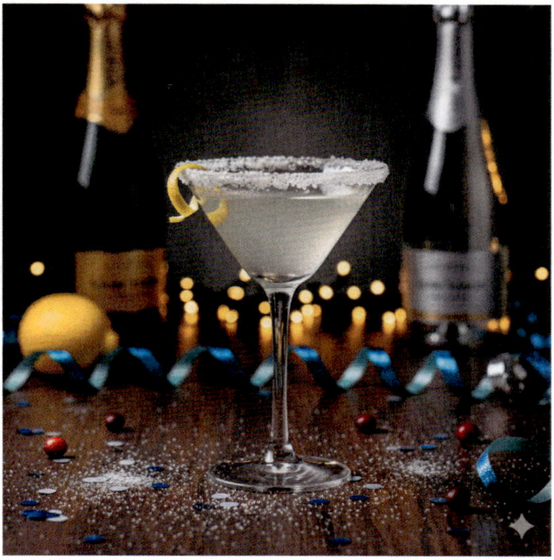

24k Margarita

2 oz Anejo Tequila

2 oz Lime Juice

1 oz Agave

½ oz Orange Juice

Grand Marnier

Edible Gold Flakes

**Add anejo tequila, lime juice, agave, orange juice, and edible gold flakes into a cocktail shaker with ice. Shake for a couple of seconds. Pour contents into a salt or sugared rimmed rocks glass with ice. Slightly pour Grand Marnier to float.

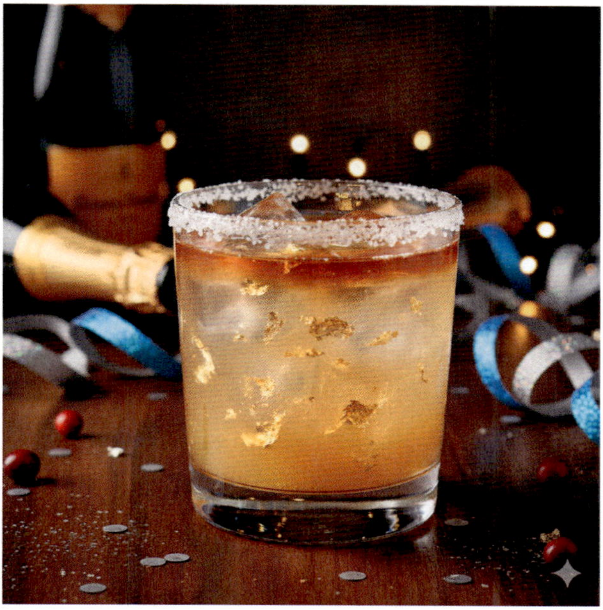

Sip of Resolution (Serves 6)

1 Cup of Strawberry Puree

4 cups of Ginger Ale

1 Bottle of champagne

1 Cup of Triple Sec

½ Cup of Lime Juice

**Add all ingredients to a large pitcher with ice. Stir gently. Serve is rocks glass with ice. Garnish with strawberries.

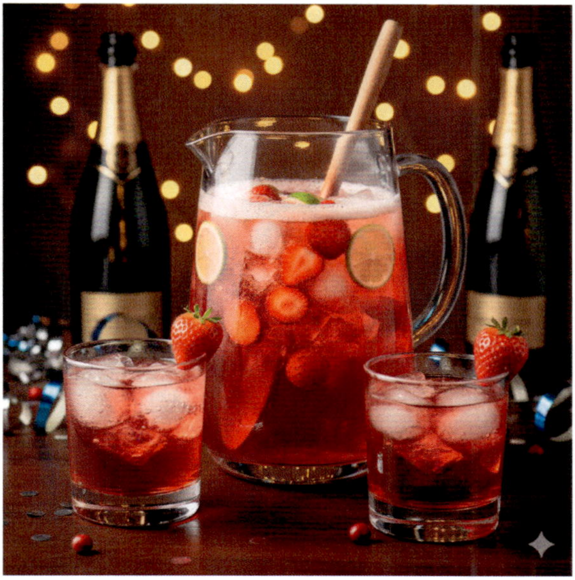

A Thank You From Me

Thank you for reaching the end of this book and sharing a little piece of your holiday season with me. I poured my heart into these pages — the memories, the recipes, the moments that shaped me — and knowing you're here means more than I can explain.

This project represents a full-circle moment in my life. After having my baby, postpartum took me through emotions and challenges I never expected. I didn't feel like myself for a long time. I questioned my confidence, my creativity, my purpose. The things I used to love felt far away, and stepping back into content creation felt almost impossible. But slowly, I started rebuilding. I started choosing myself again. And piece by piece, the spark came back.

Quitting my job was one of the scariest decisions I've ever made. But it also became the moment I realized how strong I really am. It forced me to trust my gifts, to back my dreams, and to bet on myself in a way I never had before. Creating this book reminded me that I'm capable, creative, and meant to share my voice with the world.

So thank you — for reading, for supporting, for being part of this new chapter with me. Thank you for allowing me to blend my memories with my passion for cocktails and storytelling. I hope these recipes bring comfort, joy, and a little sparkle to your holidays. I hope my stories remind you to honor your own journey, even the messy parts. And most of all, I hope you walk away believing in yourself a little more deeply too.

Here's to healing, to growth, to choosing yourself, and to celebrating every version of who you've been along the way.

With Love,

Tati

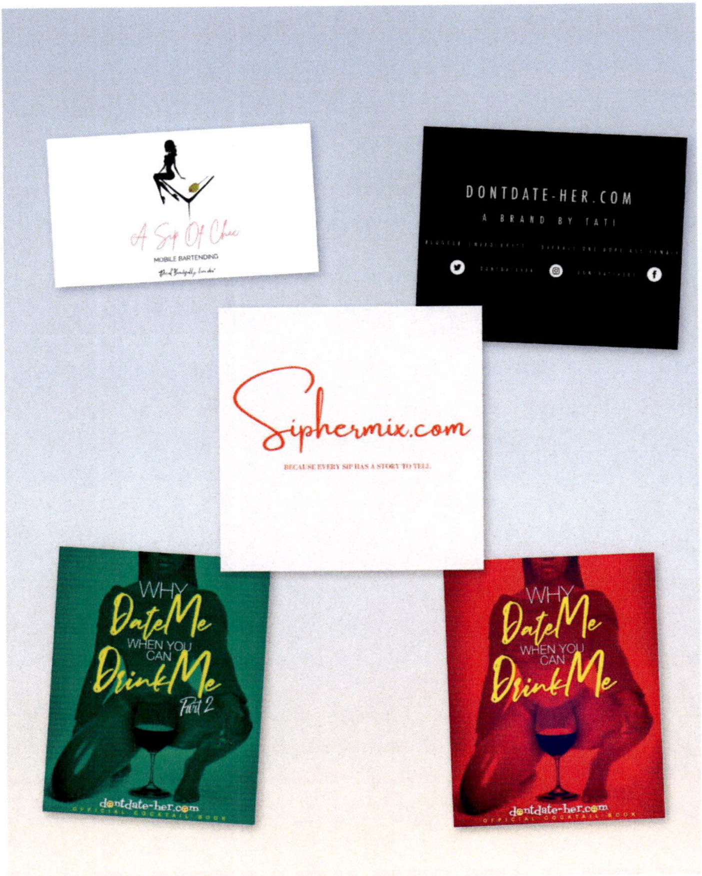
A Sip Of Chic
MOBILE BARTENDING
DONTDATE-HER.COM
A BRAND BY TATI
Siphermix.com
BECAUSE EVERY SIP HAS A STORY TO TELL.
WHY DateMe WHEN YOU CAN DrinkMe
Part 2
dontdate-her.com
OFFICIAL COCKTAIL BOOK
WHY DateMe WHEN YOU CAN DrinkMe
dontdate-her.com
OFFICIAL COCKTAIL BOOK

I GO BY TATI....

Connect *with* Me!

Siphermix.com

BECAUSE EVERY SIP HAS A STORY TO TELL

Instagram
@dontdateher1

TikTOk
@dontdateher1

YouTube
@dontdateher1

Thank You

Thank Your For Your Support !

Made in United States
Orlando, FL
04 November 2026

90202062R00048